The Holistic Twin Pregnancy Bible

A Comprehensive Approach

Copyright Page

About the Author: Julia Brooks

Julia Brooks is a dedicated health and wellness advocate, passionate about supporting women through the unique journey of twin pregnancy. With a background in holistic health and prenatal care, Julia combines her expertise and personal experiences to guide expectant mothers in nurturing their physical and emotional well-being. Her compassionate approach and commitment to empowering women have inspired many to embrace the joys and challenges of motherhood. When not writing, Julia enjoys yoga, spending time in nature, and connecting with her family. She resides in the United States (Winnipeg) where she continues her work in women's health and wellness.

Table of contents

Copyright Page

About the Author: Julia Brooks

Table of contents

Personal Story: Embracing a Medicinal Approach for a Healthy Twin Pregnancy

Stories from Twin Moms: Embracing a Holistic Journey

Bonus

Interactive Elements

Chapter 1

Foundations of Twin Pregnancy

Immediate Steps for a Healthy Start

Chapter 2

First Trimester Essentials

Personal Reflections

Chapter 3

Holistic Health Practices

Tips for Safe Prenatal Exercise:

Chapter 4

Choosing Your Medical Team for Twin Pregnancy

Chapter 5

Third Trimester Of Twins Pregnancy: full Guide

How Many Calories Should I Eat During the Third Trimester?

Twin Pregnancy Sleep Tips

Dealing with Pain in Third Trimester Pregnancy

Chapter 6

Preparing for Childbirth

Basic Advice for Preparing for Childbirth

Chapter 7: Labor, Delivery, and Beyond

How Your Twin Will Arrive + My Twin Birth Story

Typical Week of Twin Birth

What Is the Length of a Twin's Birth?

How to use essential oils for an easier home birth

Chapter 8

Postpartum Recovery and Care

Caring for Your Twins

How to Survive Newborn Twins

Chapter 10

How To Tell Identical Twins Apart

Conclusion

Glossary of Terms

Frequently Asked Questions (FAQs)

Personal Story: Embracing a Medicinal Approach for a Healthy Twin Pregnancy

Thank you for visiting "The Holistic Twin Pregnancy Bible: A Comprehensive Approach." It gives me great pleasure to set out on this amazing journey with you. I know the range of feelings and difficulties that accompany learning you are expecting two happy little bundles of joy because I am a mother of twins. This book is designed to be your go-to resource for holistic thoughts and useful advice on how to have a happy, healthy, and balanced twin pregnancy.

You'll discover a lot of material based on holistic medicine as well as medical expertise throughout these pages. The intention is to help you nurture your body, mind, and spirit in addition to your baby. This book tries to offer thorough support at every stage, whether you're adjusting to life with your twins, navigating the early weeks, or getting ready for birth.

My mind was racing with questions, fear, and joy when I found out I was carrying twins. I wanted to make sure I did everything in my power to keep my babies and myself safe and healthy because I was aware that having twins presented its own special set of dangers and challenges.

Deciding to adopt a balanced strategy that blended conventional medical care with holistic approaches was one of the most important choices I ever made. The first step in this trip was to locate a medical professional who specialized in twin pregnancies. Dr. Emily Roberts, my obstetrician, was a skilled and kind medical practitioner who recognized my wish for a comprehensive pregnant experience.

Dr. Roberts stressed the value of routine prenatal checkups and thorough screenings from the very first consultation. These health examinations were essential for tracking my twins' development and progress as well as for seeing any possible issues early on. I was very comforted by the thorough ultrasounds, which showed me my babies growing and moving.

Dr. Roberts was aware of the importance of holistic wellbeing in promoting a safe pregnancy, though. She put me in touch with a pregnant nutritionist, who assisted me in creating a diet plan full of vital nutrients specifically for twin pregnancies. It became routine to include foods high in calcium, iron, and folic acid. I also started using herbal teas and natural supplements, although I always did so with my medical team's advice.

Another essential component of my holistic approach was exercise. Swimming and gentle pregnant yoga became my go-to workouts. I was able to maintain my physical fitness and get much-needed rest and clarity of mind from these activities. During labor, the breathing exercises I had learned in yoga proved to be really helpful in helping me stay focused and control my pain.

Stress reduction was also crucial. I was urged by Dr. Roberts to routinely practice mindfulness and meditation. Even with the unavoidable worries of a twin pregnancy, I was able to maintain my composure and composure by making time each day for guided meditations and deep breathing techniques.

The network of support I created for myself was one of the journey's most remarkable features. Having a network of support, whether it be from friends and family or online twin parenting forums, makes all the difference. It was really consoling to have a sense of community among other twin moms as they shared stories, advice, and supportive remarks.

The mix of comprehensive medical care and holistic techniques provided me confidence and peace of mind as my due date drew near. Despite being incredibly stressful, my labor and delivery went well when the time came. The medical staff was equipped to handle any situation, and I felt strong and resilient because of my own comprehensive preparation.

In retrospect, I am appreciative of the well-rounded strategy that included both medical and natural methods. It guaranteed my twins' and my health and safety on the trip. This book is a mirror of that experience, providing you with a thorough manual to help you navigate the health, harmony, and confidence of your own twin pregnancy. Greetings on your incredible adventure. It's a privilege to participate in it with you.

Stories from Twin Moms: Embracing a Holistic Journey

Sarah

Sarah was ecstatic to learn she was carrying twins, but she was also intimidated by the difficulties that might arise. In an attempt to ensure a seamless pregnancy, she adopted a comprehensive strategy emphasizing diet and mindfulness.

Sarah started her daily routine with mindfulness meditation right away. She meditated for twenty minutes every morning, concentrating on her breathing and envisioning a safe pregnancy. She was able to stay composed and stress- and anxiety-free because to this practice.

Sarah not only practiced mindfulness but also developed a customized meal plan with a dietitian. She consumed a diet high in nutrients and full of the vitamins and minerals needed for twin pregnancies. Her go-to breakfast of choice was now smoothies loaded with berries, chia seeds, and leafy greens, which gave her the nutrition and energy she needed.

Sarah's all-encompassing strategy worked. She felt strong and well the entire time, and her pregnancy developed without any problems. Sarah remained composed and focused during the delivery by using the breathing exercises she had practiced as part of her meditation practice. She exuded contentment and serenity as she welcomed her twins into the world.

Emma

Emma began her journey with the twins by resolving to maintain an active lifestyle and use natural medicines to support her health. She joined up for a prenatal yoga session meant especially for expectant mothers of numerous children. In addition to keeping her physically healthy, the mild stretches and strength-training activities reduced frequent aches and pains including back pain and edema.

Emma was also introduced to the idea of herbal medicines by her yoga instructor. Emma started consuming red raspberry leaf tea, which is beneficial for fortifying the uterine muscles, as advised by her doctor. She also used essential oil of lavender to help her relax and sleep better.

Emma discovered that her life had a harmonious balance as a result of her comprehensive approach. Her supportive network of other expectant mothers was fostered by the yoga sessions, and the herbal treatments offered her a natural means of addressing pregnancy issues. Emma felt strong and self-assured after her twins were delivered since she had taken care of her body and mind the entire pregnancy.

Olivia

Olivia's twin pregnancy was characterized by a thoughtful balancing act between conventional medical care and alternative therapies. She selected a midwife who would both closely monitor the twins' development and support her wish for a natural birth.

Olivia underwent frequent acupuncture treatments as part of her holistic quest to aid with her nausea and enhance her general health. She also engaged in the practice of hypnobirthing, which is a method of controlling labor pain with self-hypnosis and relaxation. Olivia was able to maintain a connection to her body and her children because to these techniques.

Olivia followed her midwife's advise to the letter and attended all of her doctor's appointments in addition to her holistic practices. This combination made sure that any possible problems were discovered quickly and dealt with efficiently.

Olivia experienced a lengthy but tolerable labor when it came time to give birth. Her midwife's assistance was crucial, and she managed to remain composed and focused by using her hypnobirthing techniques. Olivia had a great sense of relief and thankfulness for her well-rounded approach after giving birth to her twins naturally.

Tale 4: Mia's Spiritual and Emotional Development

Mia's spiritual and emotional practices served as the foundation for her holistic journey. When she found out she was expecting twins, a lot of worries and anxiety surfaced, so she looked for strategies to support her mental health.

Mia started going to a support group for mothers of numerous children once a week. She felt less alone and more understood after talking about her experiences and listening to other people. She also began keeping a daily journal in which she wrote down her ideas and emotions, giving her emotions a constructive outlet.

Mia took spiritual comfort from her faith. She found courage and consolation in her daily regimen, which included prayer and spiritual reading. She also wrote down three things for which she was grateful each day, which helped her turn her attention from her problems to her blessings.

After the twins arrived safely, Mia felt emotionally ready to take on the tasks that lay ahead. She had a solid foundation thanks to her holistic approach, and she kept using these techniques to gracefully and resiliently handle the early stages of parenthood.

These tales demonstrate the various ways that twin mothers have adopted complementary therapies to aid in their pregnancies. All mothers' journeys are different, reflecting their own needs and preferences, but they all aim to nourish their bodies, brains, and spirits in preparation for a happy and successful twin pregnancy.

Bonus

Interactive Elements

- Journal entries
- Self-care checklists
- Questions for your doctor
- Labor visualization exercises
- Postpartum care plans
- Milestone trackers
- Resource directories
- Future goals reflection

Chapter 1

Foundations of Twin Pregnancy

Immediate Steps for a Healthy Start

Discovering that you're expecting twins is an incredible moment filled with excitement, wonder, and a flurry of questions. The first steps you take can set the tone for a healthy and positive journey through your twin pregnancy. Embracing a holistic approach right from the beginning can help you feel empowered, supported, and balanced as you embark on this remarkable path.

The very first thing to do is to schedule your initial prenatal appointment. Contact your healthcare provider as soon as you suspect or confirm a twin pregnancy. Early and regular prenatal care is essential for monitoring the health of both you and your babies. If possible, choose a healthcare provider who specializes in twin pregnancies. Their expertise can provide invaluable insights and reassurance throughout your journey.

At your first appointment, your provider will likely perform an ultrasound to confirm the twin pregnancy and check for vital signs and overall health of the babies. This early visit sets the foundation for your prenatal care schedule, which will include more frequent check-ups than with a singleton pregnancy to ensure that everything progresses smoothly.

Nutrition plays a pivotal role in a healthy twin pregnancy. Your body needs extra nutrients to support the growth and development of two babies. Begin by focusing on a balanced diet rich in essential vitamins and minerals. Include plenty of fruits, vegetables, whole grains, lean proteins, and healthy fats in your meals. Consider consulting a prenatal nutritionist who can help you create a tailored meal plan that meets the increased nutritional demands of a twin pregnancy. Staying hydrated is equally important, so make sure to drink plenty of water throughout the day.

Incorporating gentle physical activity into your routine can help you maintain strength, flexibility, and overall wellbeing. Prenatal yoga and swimming are excellent choices for expecting mothers of twins. These activities not only keep you physically fit but also promote relaxation and mental clarity. Always consult with your healthcare provider before starting any new exercise regimen to ensure it's safe for you and your babies.

Stress management is another crucial aspect of a holistic approach to twin pregnancy. The news of expecting twins can bring a mix of emotions, from joy to anxiety. Finding effective ways to manage stress can make a significant difference in your overall experience. Techniques such as mindfulness, meditation, and deep breathing exercises can help you stay calm and centered. Consider setting aside time each day for these practices, even if it's just a few minutes of quiet reflection.

Building a strong support network is essential. Reach out to family and friends and let them know about your twin pregnancy. Their encouragement and assistance can be incredibly valuable. Joining a support group for parents of multiples, either locally or online, can also provide a sense of community and shared understanding. Connecting with other twin moms who have gone through similar experiences can offer practical advice and emotional support.

Herbal remedies and natural supplements, under the guidance of your healthcare provider, can also contribute to a holistic and healthy start. For example, drinking red raspberry leaf tea may help strengthen the uterine muscles, while ginger tea can alleviate nausea. Always discuss any herbal remedies or supplements with your provider to ensure they're safe for your specific situation

As you take these initial steps, remember to listen to your body and trust your instincts. Each twin pregnancy is unique, and what works best for one person might differ for another. Be open to adjusting your approach based on how you feel and the guidance of your healthcare team.

Chapter 2

First Trimester Essentials

Regardless of the kind of twin pregnancy you are experiencing, there are a few things you should know about them right away.

Beyond fraternal and identical twins, there are three primary kinds of identical twins. However, there are more than just these two types of twins. Monochorionic Monoamniotic (MoMo), Dichorionic Diamniotic (DiDi) Twins, and Monochorionic Diamniotic (MoDi) Twins

Words that I was unfamiliar with before being pregnant with twins: Children who are neither twins or multiples are referred to as singletons by their twin parents. Consequently, a lady carrying a single child is said to be carrying a singleton pregnancy.

My Three Best Pregnancy Advice Pieces

#1 Have faith in your instincts

My best piece of advice for you during your twin pregnancy is to follow your mother's instincts. Only YOU are aware of your emotions and the wellbeing of the infants. My twins and I might not be here today if I hadn't followed my instincts as a mother.

Call the nurse line provided by your care provider or visit the hospital to get checked out if you sense something is "off."

#2 Conduct independent study

Yes, I am aware that the internet is full of false information, but if I hadn't done my own research before being pregnant with the MoDi twins, I never would have received the treatment I required when I needed it. My OBGYN was excellent during my singleton pregnancy, however he was unaware that by the time I was 16 weeks pregnant with twins, I needed to be sent to a perinatal physician or maternal fetal medicine care provider due to my high risk twin pregnancy.

#3 Speak out for your twins and yourself.

It is imperative that, after conducting thorough research, you stand up for both yourself and your twins.

Symptoms of a Twin Pregnancy

Human chorionic gonadotropin (HCG) levels are likely to be higher during twin pregnancies, which contributes to the fact that twin pregnancy symptoms are frequently more severe than singleton pregnancy symptoms.

Pregnancy symptoms differed between my twin pregnancy and my singleton pregnancy; the former's symptoms appeared considerably sooner in the first trimester and were more severe.

First Trimester Conception of Twins

Compared to the remainder of your pregnancy, the first trimester of a twin pregnancy will involve the fewest appointments. This is due to the likelihood that your first ultrasound, which will occur at 8 or 9 weeks pregnant, may reveal if you are having twins.

Depending on how informed your healthcare physician or OBGYN is about high-risk twin pregnancies and the specific type of twins you are carrying, there may be a steep learning curve at this stage. You will have fewer appointments if you are expecting fraternal twins as opposed to identical twins who share a placenta, MoDi, or MoMo twins.

Your first appointment may be at 4 weeks when you take a home pregnancy test and discover you are pregnant, or it may be at 8 weeks when you have your first ultrasound, depending on whether you were actively trying to get pregnant or if you had any preexisting issues.

Human chorionic gonadotropin (HCG) levels may be measured with blood testing during the initial prenatal visit. If you have a thyroid condition, as I do, blood tests may be performed to see whether you require further thyroid replacement.

Supplements and Diet for Holistic Expectant Mothers

A comprehensive strategy for maternal health begins with proper nutrition during pregnancy, particularly when the mother is carrying twins. Eating for two isn't enough; you also need to feed your infants and yourself a range of healthful foods that encourage healthy development and growth while enhancing your general wellbeing.

A rainbow of fruits and vegetables is the first step towards a healthy twin pregnancy diet. These offer vital vitamins, minerals, and antioxidants that are needed for immune system support and cellular operation. Add leafy greens, such as kale and spinach, which are high in iron and folate and can help avoid neural tube abnormalities and promote the creation of red blood cells.

For fetal development and mother tissue repair, lean proteins like those found in fish, chicken, lentils, and tofu are essential. They give your twins the amino acids needed to create cells and enzymes, supporting their healthy development. To lessen your exposure to hazardous substances, choose sources that are low in saturated fats and, if at all possible, seek organic ones.

Complex carbs found in whole grains like quinoa, brown rice, and oats provide you long-lasting energy and vital elements like fiber, magnesium, and B vitamins. These nutrients support healthy digestion, which can change during pregnancy, and help control blood sugar levels.

Avocados, nuts, seeds, and olive oil are good sources of healthy fats that are crucial for the development of the fetus's brain and the synthesis of hormones by the mother. Flaxseeds, walnuts, and fatty fish like salmon are good sources of omega-3 fatty acids, which support a baby's developing brain and eyes.

Staying hydrated is important during pregnancy, especially if you are expecting twins. Water facilitates nutrition transfer, aids in digestion and circulation, and maintains amniotic fluid levels. Aim for eight to ten glasses a day, more or less depending on your needs and degree of exercise.

A comprehensive pregnancy nutrition plan include supplements as a supplementary element. Prenatal vitamins, designed especially for expectant moms, guarantee sufficient consumption of folic acid, iron, calcium, and other vital elements that may be difficult to get from diet alone. Talk to your doctor about tailoring your supplement regimen to your specific needs depending on your blood tests.

Probiotics can help with digestion and immune system function by fostering gut health. Yogurt, kefir, and fermented foods like kimchi and sauerkraut are examples of natural sources. It could also be advised to take probiotic supplements to keep the proper balance of gut flora.

Herbal remedies, including ginger tea, can ease the usual pregnant symptoms of nausea and upset stomach. But before using any herbal remedies or supplements, proceed with caution and get advice from your healthcare professional. Some of them may interfere with pharmaceuticals or put your pregnancy at risk.

In addition to promoting the health and development of your unborn children, adopting a comprehensive approach to nutrition and supplementation during your twin pregnancy can also improve your own wellbeing. Pay attention to what your body needs, get advice from medical professionals, and embrace this life-changing experience with vigor and confidence.

Holistic Meal and Supplement Plan for Pregnant Woman with Twins

Breakfast:

- **Smoothie**: Blend spinach, kale, frozen berries, banana, Greek yogurt, and flaxseed meal with almond milk.

- **Whole Grain Toast**: Top with avocado and a sprinkle of chia seeds.

Mid-Morning Snack:

- **Mixed Nuts**: Almonds, walnuts, and cashews.
- **Fruit**: Apple slices with almond butter.

Lunch:

- **Quinoa Salad**: Mixed greens, cooked quinoa, chickpeas, cherry tomatoes, cucumber, and feta cheese with olive oil and lemon dressing.

- **Side**: Whole grain crackers with hummus.

Afternoon Snack:

- **Greek Yogurt**: Plain yogurt with honey and mixed berries.
- **Trail Mix**: Dried apricots, pumpkin seeds, and dark chocolate chips.

Dinner:

- **Grilled Salmon**: Serve with roasted sweet potatoes and steamed broccoli.

- **Side**: Quinoa pilaf with spinach and pine nuts.

Evening Snack:

- **Homemade Popcorn**: Air-popped with a sprinkle of nutritional yeast and sea salt.
- **Herbal Tea**: Chamomile or ginger tea for relaxation.

Supplements:

- **Prenatal Vitamin**: Ensure it includes folic acid, iron, calcium, vitamin D, and omega-3 fatty acids.
- **Probiotics**: Support digestive health and immunity.
- **Additional Supplements**: As recommended by healthcare provider based on individual needs, such as vitamin B12 or magnesium.

Hydration:

- **Water**: Drink at least 8-10 glasses per day.
- **Infused Water**: Add slices of citrus fruits or cucumber for added flavor.

Notes:

- **Balanced Intake**: Ensure meals include a balance of proteins, healthy fats, complex carbohydrates, and fiber.

- **Variety**: Incorporate a variety of colorful fruits and vegetables to maximize nutrient intake.

- **Cooking Methods**: Opt for grilling, baking, or steaming over frying to retain nutrients.

- **Consultation**: Always consult with a healthcare provider or nutritionist to tailor the plan to individual needs and ensure safety and effectiveness throughout the pregnancy journey.

Interactive: Personal Diary

- Space for readers to track symptoms and feelings

- **Symptoms**

- **Weight**

- **Medications**

Personal Reflections*:*

- **Challenges**: Document any challenges you're facing and how you're coping with them.

- **Joys**: Write about special moments or achievements during your pregnancy.

- **Gratitude**: List things you're grateful for

Chapter 3

Holistic Health Practices

Physical Wellness: Safe Exercises for Twin Pregnancies

Maintaining physical wellness during a twin pregnancy is crucial for your overall health and the well-being of your babies. While exercise is beneficial, it's important to choose activities that are safe and supportive of your changing body. Here's a look at safe exercises tailored for twin pregnancies:

1. Walking: A low-impact exercise that you can easily incorporate into your daily routine. Walking helps improve circulation, maintain cardiovascular health, and boost your mood without putting excessive strain on your joints.

2. Swimming: Ideal for expectant mothers of twins as it provides a full-body workout while reducing the impact on your joints. Swimming helps strengthen muscles, improves flexibility, and promotes relaxation, which can be particularly soothing during pregnancy.

3. Prenatal Yoga: Specifically designed yoga poses and sequences tailored to the needs of pregnant women can help improve flexibility, balance, and circulation. Prenatal yoga also emphasizes breathing techniques that can aid in relaxation and prepare you for labor.

4. Modified Strength Training: Light resistance exercises using body weight, resistance bands, or light weights can help maintain muscle tone and strength. Focus on exercises that target major muscle groups while avoiding exercises that strain your abdominal muscles excessively.

5. Pelvic Floor Exercises (Kegels): Strengthening your pelvic floor muscles can help prevent urinary incontinence and prepare you for childbirth. These exercises involve contracting and relaxing the muscles around your bladder and vagina.

Yoga and Prenatal Fitness Routines

Prenatal Yoga: Prenatal yoga is specifically adapted for the changes your body goes through during pregnancy, particularly with twins. It focuses on gentle stretching, breathing exercises, and relaxation techniques. These practices can help alleviate common pregnancy discomforts, such as back pain and swelling, while promoting emotional well-being.

Benefits of Prenatal Yoga:

- **Improved Flexibility:** Helps maintain flexibility and range of motion in joints, which can become stiff due to hormonal changes.

- **Stress Reduction:** Incorporates mindfulness and deep breathing techniques that promote relaxation and reduce stress levels.

- **Connection with Baby:** Provides a calm and nurturing environment for you to bond with your babies as you become more aware of their movements and presence.

Prenatal Fitness Routines: In addition to yoga, incorporating other forms of prenatal fitness can further enhance your physical well-being. These routines are designed to be gentle yet effective, supporting your body as it undergoes the demands of carrying twins.

Tips for Safe Prenatal Exercise:

- **Consult with Your Healthcare Provider:** Before starting any exercise program, discuss your plans with your healthcare provider to ensure it's safe for your pregnancy and individual health needs.

- **Listen to Your Body:** Pay attention to how your body feels during exercise. If you experience discomfort, dizziness, or shortness of breath, stop and rest.

- **Stay Hydrated:** Drink plenty of water before, during, and after exercise to stay hydrated.

- **Avoid Overexertion:** Choose exercises that are moderate in intensity and avoid activities that involve lying flat on your back or require sudden changes in direction.

Interactive diary session

Checklist – Tick beside the done tasks

- Attend prenatal appointments regularly
- Take prenatal vitamins as prescribed.
- Stay hydrated by drinking enough water.
- Eat a balanced diet rich in fruits, vegetables, and whole grains.
- Engage in safe physical activities approved by your healthcare provider.
- Get sufficient rest and sleep.
- Practice self-care and relaxation techniques.

Chapter 4

Choosing Your Medical Team for Twin Pregnancy

Choosing your medical team for a twin pregnancy is one of the first things you should do once you see those two little dots on your first ultrasound. Even if you've been pregnant before, you probably know that twin pregnancies sometimes needs extra care and consideration. As such, choosing the best medical team for you and your twins should be one of your top priorities in the coming weeks. If you're unsure about how to choose or need to know more, we've got you covered. Here's everything you need to know about choosing the best medical team for your twin pregnancy.

Why Do I Need a Medical Team for My Twin Pregnancy?

The main distinction between a twin pregnancy, aside from the larger bulge and a few more doctor's appointments, is the higher chance of difficulties for both the mother and the unborn child. The most crucial elements of a successful twin pregnancy are the prevention, observation, and management of these issues. A varied medical team can help guarantee the safest and healthiest outcome for everyone, even though many twin pregnancies go really well with just one care provider.

Your risk of problems is influenced by your medical history, prior pregnant experience, and the outcomes of any prenatal screenings or tests. Among the difficulties are:

Pre-eclampsia

hypertension during pregnancy (high blood pressure)

Diabetes during pregnancy

Anemia

Problems with fetal development

Previa placenta

premature delivery

early birth

section by cesarean

bleeding after giving birth

Your risk factors and the type of care you receive will also be influenced by the type of twins you are having. Pregnancies involving dichorionic-diagmniotic (Di-Di) twins—most often, fraternal twins—are typically lower risk and offer more options for prenatal care.

Having identical twins makes things a little trickier right away. Monochorionic-Diamniotic kids, often known as Mo-Di or Mono-Di, have a thin membrane separating the babies from the placenta. Monochorionic-Monoamniotic, often known as Mo-Mo or Mono-Mono, share the amniotic sac and placenta. Sharing is wonderful, but having a single placenta exposes them to all of those risks in addition to issues unique to identical twins, like:

Syndrome of Twin-to-Twin Transfusion (TTTS)

The selective intrauterine growth restriction known as selective twin anemia polycythemia sequence (TAPS) (sIUGR)

Even while many twin pregnancies end well, problems can arise at any time, and twin pregnancies frequently necessitate the assistance of a larger medical team for intervention and support.

A doctor from the woman's medical care team examines her during her pregnancy.

How Should I Select My Twin Pregnancy Medical Team?

Your comfort level and the medical team's experience are the most important factors to take into account. Your ideal medical team should be able to provide numerous types of care and delivery while also making you feel comfortable and secure in their abilities. Steer clear of any professional who tries to minimize your worries or who thinks there are no differences between a twin pregnancy and a singleton pregnancy.

If you are expecting twins, you may want to see the obstetrician or midwife you have previously seen. All right, this is good to hear, but make sure you ask about their twin experience—pregnancy, labor, and delivery included. Find out about their twin delivery experiences, including any issues they had to deal with. Do they possess prior experience delivering a double-whammy? What happens if something arises that they are ill-prepared to deal with? Take the time to interview potential new healthcare providers if your current one is unable to manage your twin pregnancy.

The hospital credentials held by your provider are a crucial factor to take into account. During and after labor, twins may need particular care, even if your provider provides the greatest prenatal care. Time spent in the Neonatal Intensive Care Unit (NICU) is frequently included in this. Because of this, a physician with privileges in a hospital with at least a Level II NICU should always be a part of your medical team.

You may frequently be restricted to what is readily available in your location, particularly in rural areas. Make sure your prenatal care and delivery are handled by a professional who can handle twins, or be ready to travel. Investigate social programs that facilitate high-risk pregnant women's access to prenatal care if this is the case.

Interview every healthcare professional in your area throughout the first few weeks of your pregnancy to choose who best suits your needs. The most crucial member of your team will give birth to your twins and handle prenatal care. Various solutions are available to you based on your pregnancy's need.

Obstetrician (OB)

A physician who specializes in treating patients during pregnancy, labor, and delivery is known as an obstetrician (OB). In addition to offering gynecological care, they also treat women both before and after childbirth. OBs go through a rigorous educational program that includes four years of medical school and a bachelor's degree. After that, students spend four years in a residency program where doctors receive practical training in diagnosing, treating, and attending births.

To keep an eye on your health as well as the health of your twins, OBs utilize a variety of instruments, including ultrasounds, prenatal screenings and testing, blood and urine tests. In addition to being adept at giving birth in a variety of settings, they frequently enjoy special access to hospitals that offer neonatal critical care. As one of the greatest options for a safe and healthy twin pregnancy, OBs are extremely qualified.

midwife

A midwife is a qualified medical practitioner who offers a variety of prenatal, postpartum, and other women's health services and support. Although midwives have a variety of qualifications and experiences, most of them emphasize more natural childbirth and pregnancy. For a safe and straightforward twin pregnancy, a certified nurse midwife can offer prenatal and delivery care; ideally, this can happen at a hospital or birth center.

However, many midwives are unable or unwilling to deliver twins alone due to the higher likelihood of problems necessitating hospital assistance. Legal limitations exist in certain states regarding midwives attending twin births in the absence of a doctor. Nevertheless, a midwife can still be a very valuable member of your medical team. They provide labor assistance and prenatal care and frequently collaborate with an OB or MFM. In addition, midwives counsel and encourage expectant parents and, if necessary, stand up for mothers and infants.

Expert in Maternal Fetal Monitoring

One particular kind of obstetrician trained to treat high-risk pregnancies, such as twins and higher order multiples, is a Maternal Fetal Monitoring expert (MFM). They acquire further training and become capable of managing a wide range of challenges.

Contrary to popular assumption, seeing an MFM is not a must when you are pregnant with twins. Instead, they are a choice if difficulties or increased risk factors throughout your pregnancy necessitate further support.

Comprehensive monitoring is offered by an MFM, which includes diagnostic testing like as amniocentesis and chorionic villus testing, as well as ultrasounds to detect growth and fluids. An MFM can manage all of your pregnancy and delivery care, even though they are typically called upon to handle issues and coordinate treatment with your prenatal care provider.

Adding Members to Your Twin Pregnancy Medical Team

You can add more resources to your medical team after selecting your prenatal care providers in order to have the healthiest possible pregnancy.

Assistant

A doula assists the person giving birth by attending to their physical and emotional needs throughout labor and delivery, as opposed to provide medical treatment. Among the many services that doulas offer is encouragement to speak up for oneself and one's birthing choices. In addition to providing information on labor and delivery techniques, a doula can perform therapeutic interventions such massage, aromatherapy, and acupressure.

Try to start the procedure as soon as possible if you decide to include a doula in your group. Set up several meetings with them to discuss your birthing plan, including their part on the day of delivery, and to strengthen your bond.

Remember that even with a flawless pregnancy, twin labor can be unpredictable and necessitate surgery. Your doula might not be able to come if you require an emergency C-section. Hospital operating room capacity limits are frequently to blame for this. Before committing, make sure to find out from your hospital whether your doula is permitted to be in the operating room. To locate a doula close to you, visit DONA.org.

When expecting twins, a doula can be a huge help to your medical team.

Counselor for Genetics

A healthy pregnancy includes prenatal genetic testing and screening. A genetic counselor assists families at every step of fertility and postpartum care by managing all facets of risk assessment, testing, and diagnosis. A genetic counselor can assist you in understanding and preparing for the birth of your child if they have been diagnosed with or are at risk for a chromosomal anomaly or defect. They can also help you with care planning and treatment options.

Dietitian

Eating for three may seem like a terrific idea—after all, no one can criticize you—but meeting your body's nutritional demands while also caring for two infants is not always simple. Making the finest food decisions to satisfy your daily nutritional demands might be assisted by a nutritionist. To maximize your intake, they might offer meal plans and supplement recommendations. Specific issues like excessive blood pressure and gestational diabetes can also be addressed by a dietitian. Make sure to consult a dietitian if you're struggling to control your food.

Consultant for Lacatation

The assistance of a lactation consultant (LC) will probably be beneficial if you choose to breastfeed your twins. When issues emerge, lactation counselors (LCs) can give solutions and invaluable support, including information about breastfeeding twins. LCs are typically employed by hospitals and NICUs, but you may also hire one yourself—Natalie Diaz from Twiniversity is one such example.

Doula for Postpartum

The actual work has only just begun, as if giving birth to twins and surviving them were not difficult enough. Parents might receive many forms of care from a postpartum doula during the postpartum period. This covers assistance with nursing, psychological and physical healing, baby care methods, and easier access to neighborhood resources. Some even offer more direct care, such meal preparation, light housekeeping, running errands, and looking after siblings (and what mother wouldn't appreciate that kind of assistance?). By hiring a postpartum doula, you and your spouse may concentrate on attending to the needs of your newborns.

As a member of their medical team throughout pregnancy, a doctor poses in front of her pregnant patient and her spouse.

When selecting your medical team for a twin pregnancy, take your time.

Even if you find out on a subsequent scan, learning you are expecting twins can completely upend your world. However, the availability of information, testing, medical assistance, and support can significantly impact your experience. Selecting your medical team will be one of the most crucial decisions you make in the upcoming months, among many others. Take your time, look into your alternatives, and select medical professionals who have experience with twins and who will make you feel supported during your twin pregnancy.

Interactive session

You can ask your doctor questions.

Think back on your pregnant experience and any questions you may have as you get ready for your upcoming doctor's visit. Use these discussion starters to help you get started:

Recognizing Your Expectancy:

How are my twins' growth and development coming along in comparison to a pregnancy with a singleton?

What significant turning points or indicators should we be watching out for during each trimester when having twins?

Health and Well-Being: What particular dietary requirements or issues should I be aware of in light of a twin pregnancy?

Do I need to take any extra vitamins or supplements to assist the development of the kids and my health?

Physical Activity: During this twin pregnancy, are there any particular exercises or physical activities that are safe and healthy for me?

How can I adjust my workout regimen to maintain efficacy and safety as my pregnancy goes on?

What are the possible difficulties or things to keep in mind before giving birth to twins?

Are there any symptoms or indicators that I should be aware of that would suggest I should visit the hospital right away?

Postpartum Care: After having twins, what should I anticipate in terms of recuperation and postpartum care?

Are mothers of multiples eligible for any special accommodations or services?

Emotional Health: How can I effectively control my stress and anxiety during my twin pregnancy?

Do you have any recommendations for services or support groups for expectant mothers of twins? This is optional.

Chapter 5

Third Trimester Of Twins Pregnancy: full Guide

When Does the Third Trimester With Twins Start?

With a single baby you will be in your third trimester from around weeks 29 or 30 through the end of your pregnancy. When it comes to a twin pregnancy, you will want to adjust this by about 2-3 weeks.

This means that **technically the third trimester with twins starts around about**

27-28 weeks. Many changes will take place during this trimester with twins, just the same as it would with one baby.

At this point in your twin pregnancy, although your babies are growing well and within a few weeks they could come into the world, it is best that they stay safe and warm in the womb as long as possible. The following topics look at the various changes your twins will go through in the third trimester before they are ready to enter the world.

How Much Will My Twins Grow During the Third Trimester?

By the third trimester in your twin pregnancy your babies would have grown quite substantially. But of course they will continue to grow even more. Twins growth during the third trimester is slower than that of their singleton counterparts.

Your twin babies organs will continue to develop and their bones will start to harden. During this third trimester of your pregnancy you may experience much higher levels of indigestion and discomfort.

You can expect to have an increase in the following symptoms due to your two babies growing more and more each week.

- Fatigue

- Pelvic pain

- Swelling

- Back pain

- Struggling to eat (with two little growing bodies in your belly there is not much room left for food)

At the start of the third trimester the average weight of twins is roughly 2.2 pounds each – so just take that into consideration when you are looking at your own weight gain. The length of each of your twins by 30 weeks is roughly 10.5 inches from crown to rump.

Will I Still Feel the Twins Moving During Third Trimester Pregnancy?

One of the biggest differences between a singleton pregnancy and a twin pregnancy is how quickly your twins will run out of room as they grow. This means that although you will still feel the twins moving during the early part of the third trimester, these movements will become less as the third trimester goes on. Additionally, you will definitely feel a lot less pronounced movements than that of a singleton pregnancy. On the other hand, you may feel more pressure pushing down on your abdomen – and of course your bladder, but the kicks and elbow jabs will be felt less often.

Many pregnant twin moms wonder if they will be able to tell the difference between each baby's movement. The truth is that unless you know for certain who is laying where, you won't really be able to tell who is delivering the kicks and jabs – especially not in the third trimester.

How Big Will My Belly Be With Twins?

We can say with all certainty that your belly will be a lot bigger than if you were just having one baby. Remember with twins, your body has to adjust and make room for two babies both trying to grow at the same speed (although it is very rare that both babies will grow at exactly the same rate throughout the pregnancy). This will mean you will pick up a lot more weight during a twin pregnancy, as well as, have a belly that measures bigger. For example, at 21 weeks of twin pregnancy your belly size is about the same as a single pregnant belly would be at 25–26 weeks.

You can keep track of the measurement of your belly at home if you want. But, rest assured your physician will do this too at every checkup.

How Much Weight Should I Gain in the Third Trimester of Twin Pregnancy?

When you are pregnant it is normal to pick up weight and in fact it is healthy to do so, but in moderation. With a twin pregnancy the amount of weight you gain will be considerably more, I mean you are having two babies, so this is to be expected.

But how much weight should you gain in the third trimester? Here is a guideline:

- Underweight (starting BMI) – aim to gain approximately 21 – 26 pounds
- Normal to overweight – aim to gain approximately 14 – 22 pounds

The next question is how much should you be gaining on a weekly basis. Again, this will depend on your unique circumstances, but a good rule of thumb is that you will gain about 1.5 pounds per week in the third trimester of twins pregnancy.

How Many Calories Should I Eat During the Third Trimester?

Now that you know how much weight you should be gaining, it's time to figure out how you are going to do this. There is actually a formula to ensure you and your babies gain weight in a healthy way.

- First Trimester – Increase calorie intake by 300 calories per baby
- Second Trimester – Increase calorie intake by 340 calories per baby

- Third Trimester – Increase by a whopping 452 calories per baby

The key to taking in a good amount of calories per day is to eat a variety of foods. Make sure you include lots of healthy fats, leafy green vegetables, protein, and carbohydrates (you need the energy after all).

Surviving The Third Trimester With Twins

Once the third trimester hits, you have come so far! But, you may be feeling like you cannot take another minute of it.

Below is our guide to help you when it comes to surviving the third trimester with twins.

Twin Pregnancy Sleep Tips

"Get as much sleep as you can before the babies arrive." Ha! That's easier said than done. By the time you hit the third trimester you may find yourself struggling more and more with sleep.

Here are some twin pregnancy sleep tips to help you through it:

- Sleep on your left side – this will be more comfortable for you and be more nourishing for your babies
- Get yourself a **body pillow**

- Develop a relaxing pregnancy bedtime routine – and stick to it
- Eat a balanced diet – avoid heavy meals too close to bed time
- Rope your spouse in for a back massage as you drift off to sleep
- Try some pregnancy yoga before you climb into bed
- Nap as much as you can

How To Deal with Exhaustion During Pregnancy

You're so tired! It is expected at this point during your pregnancy, but how can you deal with the exhaustion in a healthy way?

We have listed some tips that should help you during your last stretch of twin pregnancy.

- Limit caffeine – this should be a given, but caffeine can cause spikes of adrenalin and then cause a crash which is definitely something you want to avoid
- Exercise daily – even in your last trimester, as long as you are healthy and it is approved by your physician, continue to do mild exercises daily
- Take naps
- Eat a balanced diet to keep your energy levels boosted and sustained
- Pamper yourself often

- Relax whenever you get the chance
- Put your feet up
- Ask for help

Dealing with Pain in Third Trimester Pregnancy

As your baby bump grows in your third trimester, you will start to experience discomfort, aches, and pains that are more prevalent.

Below is a list of third trimester pregnancy pains you may feel.

- **Braxton Hicks** – these are abdominal pains that are similar to labor pains. Braxton Hicks are likened to practice contractions. The way to get through them – breathe deeply and calm your body.

- **Back & Hip Pain** – Your posture will change according to your growing bump, which will contribute to this pain. The fact that there is an increase in progesterone which softens the muscles and ligaments can also increase pain. To ease this discomfort you can use a **support belt under your belly**.

- **Round Ligament Pain** – This is probably the most common pain. It is a sharp pain felt in the lower belly and groin area. The round ligament is stretched and strained as your belly grows. The way to deal with this pain is to do lots of exercise to keep your stomach muscles strong. Do not make sudden movements and flex your hip muscles for support.

- **Pelvic Pain** – This will often be felt in the pubic bone and also causes a pressure build up on your vaginal muscles. Pelvic floor exercises to strengthen muscles can help with the pain. A prenatal massage, warm bath or shower, and rest can also help cope with this pain.

As with any pain that is persistent, if you feel that it is not easing no matter what you do, please make sure you see your physician as soon as possible to rule out any other complications.

Bed Rest With Twins

Bed rest is often recommended for high risk pregnancies or for pregnancies where a complication has been detected. In twin pregnancy bed rest is more common, purely because carrying around two babies is higher risk and comes with more complications.

If you are put on bed rest the way to cope with it is to just take it in your stride. Ask for help and accept help that is offered.

Pregnancy is tough, rewarding, and amazing, but it is especially a struggle towards the end, so take all the help you can get.

Final Preparations For Arrival of Two Newborns

You are in your final weeks before your babies arrive. So, what should you have in place in preparation for twins? Here is a basic checklist to help you on your way.

- Pack the hospital bag for babies, mom, and dad
- Get **bassinets / co-sleepers** ready

- Create a **twin birth plan** (if applicable)
- Stock up on toiletries, medical items etc.
- Meal preparation for at least the first 4 weeks
- Wash all baby clothes and blankets
- Invest in a **daily newborn twin babies tracker**

You can also do **prenatal classes** during this time, choose a pediatrician, tour the hospital, and most importantly – take care of yourself!

Pregnancy during the third trimester with twins is both an exciting and scary time. If you are struggling hang in there, it's not that much longer until you will be meeting your beautiful twin babies!

Remember that you need to take care of yourself during this time as well. Some of the main points to take away from this article are:

- Rest as much as possible
- Preparation is key
- Eat well
- Do everything in moderation
- Accept help when it is offered
- Take a **birthing class**
- ENJOY your pregnancy

Personal interactive diary session

Personal affirmation, say these and mean it

"I am strong, capable, and ready for this beautiful journey."

"My body knows how to nourish and protect my babies."

"I embrace the changes in my body with love and gratitude."

"Every day, I am more prepared to welcome my twins."

"I am surrounded by support, love, and positivity."

"I trust my instincts as a mother of twins."

"I am creating a healthy and nurturing environment for my babies."

"Each moment brings me closer to meeting my little ones."

"I am resilient and will overcome any challenges."

"My twins and I are connected through love and strength."

Chapter 6

Preparing for Childbirth

I hope you feel more equipped to handle labor and delivery with twins now that you've read my tale of vaginal induction twin birth and maybe a twin C-section birth birth as well.

The excitement and anxiety of expecting a new baby to enter the world are mutually reinforcing. A smoother and more enjoyable childbirth experience for you and your child is dependent on your level of preparation, regardless of whether you're planning a hospital birth or preferring the closeness of an at-home delivery.

Getting Ready for a Hospital Birth Package Your Medical Purse Initial requirements for you: Personal products, nursing bras, maternity pads, nursing bras, and comfortable apparel. Provide a list of crucial contacts—like family and friends—so they can be kept informed during labor.

For the infant: Outfits, covers, diapers, and any additional goods specific to the early days. Important papers including your birth plan, insurance information, and ID should not be overlooked.

Understand Hospital Procedures and Your Route

Learn the way to the hospital, particularly if it's not close by. Recognize the parking procedures, labor and delivery policies, and admissions procedures of the hospital. To acquaint yourself with the trip, think about making a trial run to the hospital.

Keep the hospital's phone number handy in case you have any last-minute questions.

Make a plan for childbirth.

Together with your healthcare practitioner, make a birth plan that details your choices for pain management, labor, delivery, and postpartum care.

Talk to your healthcare professional about backup plans in case the plan needs to be modified.

Make Travel Arrangements Make sure you have a dependable way to get to the hospital. As the deadline draws near, keep your stuff in the car or close to the entrance.

Carry a car charger and a fully charged phone in your suitcase.

Be aware of several ways to get around in case your main plan doesn't work out.

Remain knowledgeable and aware.

Take childbirth education classes to learn about the phases of labor, ways to manage pain, and how to breathe and relax during contractions.

To make connections with other expectant parents, look via internet forums and tools.

Make use of relaxation techniques in your everyday routine and practice them at home.

Getting Ready for a Home Birth

Establish a Birth Space Pick a calm, cozy location for the birth. If you want to give birth under water, think about adding features like a delivery pool, cozy seating, and enough lighting.

Incorporate relaxing components into your chosen birth area, such as aromatherapy candles or relaxing music.

Make sure your birth partner or support person has a cozy chair or mat.

Put Your Birth Kit Together

Assemble the supplies that your midwife or healthcare professional has advised. These could include of towels, sterile gloves, sterile pads, thermometers, and any other particular materials advised for the birth.

Make a checklist and check your birth kit again to make sure nothing is missed.

The birth kit should be kept in a convenient place.

Maintain a Plan B.

Have a backup plan in place in case something goes wrong, even if you are planning an at-home birth. Identify the closest hospital and arrange for transportation in case it becomes necessary.

Talk to your birth attendant in detail about the backup plan, and make sure everyone is aware of it.

Have a first aid kit on hand that is completely filled.

Make Plans for Doula or Midwife Assistance

Make sure the birth attendant you have selected is prepared with all the tools needed and is aware of the delivery plan.

In this process, communication is essential.

Ahead of your due date, arrange to see your doula or midwife on a regular basis.

To build understanding and trust with your birth team, practice good communication.

Utilize calming methods

Together with your partner or birth coach, practice breathing exercises, relaxation techniques, and labor positions. These can be quite helpful when giving birth.

Take pregnant yoga lessons to improve your flexibility and level of calmness.

To assist create a relaxing ambiance, compile a playlist of calming music.

Basic Advice for Preparing for Childbirth

Get ready Psychologically and emotionally, birth can be erratic. Learn your stuff, but also be open to having your plans altered. Remain adaptable and receptive.

To enhance emotional well–being, try mindfulness exercises like journaling or meditation.

If you want guidance and experiences from others, go to prenatal classes or support groups.

Continue to Eat and Stay Hydrated.

Eat well and drink plenty of water. Throughout labor, keep food on hand for sudden energy spikes.

Stow wholesome snacks in your hospital bag that combine carbohydrates and protein.

While in labor, keep a bottle of water close at hand.

Maintain Contact with Assistance

Establish a network of support, including your spouse, family, and friends, to help you through labor and delivery.

To guarantee a coordinated effort, talk to your support system about roles and expectations and document them.

Plan your communications so that everyone is aware of updates and information.

Maintain Vital Contacts Close at Hand

Keep a list of emergency contacts on your phone, along with the number of your healthcare practitioner and any other pertinent connections.

Put the main desk number of the hospital into your phone for non-urgent questions.

For convenient access, save a list of postpartum support resources.

Remain Calm and Believe in Yourself

Recall that your body is made for this amazing experience. Have faith in your intuition and yourself.

Prior to labor, practice affirmations that will give you confidence.

For stress relief, think about relaxation techniques or prenatal massages.

Don't forget to adjust these recommendations to your requirements and tastes. Ask your birthing team if you need any specialized advice or if you have any questions!

Interactive

Create your Worksheet for Birth Plans

Chapter 7: Labor, Delivery, and Beyond

How Your Twin Will Arrive + My Twin Birth Story

Giving birth to twins is a thrilling and terrifying experience. As much as you may be excited to meet your two tiny bundles of joy, most expectant twin parents find that becoming to that point frightening, particularly if this is their first pregnancy. I had twins for the first time. I'm sharing my birth story, lessons learned, and advice to help others who could be in a similar situation. It is my goal to assist you in preparing for the labor and delivery of your own twin pregnancy.

Please be aware that this post contains affiliate links. To find out more, see my disclosure & privacy policy at the bottom of this page.

What Makes Twin Births Unique?

When it comes to a twin pregnancy birth, the two main differences are:

Giving birth in the operation room

How many people were there when it was delivered

Giving Birth in the Operating Room

The most significant aspect of your delivery experience will be giving birth to your twins in the operating room. You will most likely be wheeled into an operating room for birth, even if you are not having a C-section.

Remember that there is a greater chance of needing to convert to a C-section if you intend to deliver your twins vaginally. Because of this, twin deliveries frequently take place in operating rooms rather than the more commonplace but nonetheless comfortable hospital labor and delivery rooms.

Attendees of the Twin Delivery

The amount of individuals in attendance for the arrival of your twins will be the second factor that has changed. Every infant will have a nurse, as well as you.

Two NICU nurses were also there because my twins were born at 35 weeks gestation. Your doctor will also be present.

Medical students might be more interested in witnessing a twin delivery. At the teaching hospital where I gave birth to my twins, a medical student completing a rotation alongside my OB/GYN worked as a resident.

You don't have to allow the medical student to be there; I consented to her being there. Fortunately, he was quite kind and ended up supporting one of my legs when I gave birth.

The anesthesiologist was also present when the baby was delivered. This was just in case a C-section needed to be performed.

Finally, but most definitely not least, my spouse was present. That means, if you're counting, there were ten people in the operating room—not counting the twins and me—during the delivery.

In contrast, with my singleton's vaginal delivery, the attending physician, her resident, a nurse for me, a nurse for the infant, and my spouse were present. That is only half of the individuals who were here when I gave birth to my twins.

How to Get Ready for the Birth of Twins

When you get to the hospital to give birth to your twins, what should you do and know? I firmly believe that attending a birthing class is quite beneficial. In addition to taking a Lamaze class for labor and delivery, you should see if your local hospital offers any classes on twin pregnancy.

The hospital provided a unique twins birth and pregnancy class that I personally attended. This is a great choice, if it's available to you.

I would have preferred to have taken a labor and delivery class as well. Regretfully, I was mistaken in my assumption that the twins class would provide ample knowledge about labor. There was some discussion about labor and delivery, but having gone through the experience of giving birth to twins, I would have rather taken a birthing class in addition.

Twins' Hospital Bag

Packing your hospital bag is another something you should do in advance. So what should you include in your bag in case you have twins?

This is what I have listed. It is best to have it ready by weeks thirty to thirty-three. Twins are known for showing up early!

Two outfits for each infant to wear on the way home

Two pairs of yoga pants or pregnancy leggings for the mother

Mom needs a cozy shirt for her trip home.

For mom, pajamas and robe

Dad's or partner's new clothes

Personal hygiene

ties for hair

Snacks: trail mix, chips, granola bars, etc.

Charger for phones

Reading material, tablets, etc.

Be Aware of These Indices of Twin Labor

How are you going to know when labor begins? There are several common indicators, and this is a good question. In the middle of the night, my water broke. I believed I had soaked the bed when I was sound sleeping. However, after it occurred once more, I discovered my water pipe was broken.

I experienced minor spotting and cramping with my singleton all day. I also experienced 18 hours of contractions spaced roughly 10 to 20 minutes apart.

<u>Typical Week of Twin Birth</u>

Given that you are expecting twins, you are probably aware of the general birthdate difference between twins and singletons. Furthermore, there is an increased chance of preterm labor during a twin pregnancy.

Plan to give birth to your twins by 38 weeks. The majority of doctors won't let a twin pregnancy proceed past this stage. Twins are often delivered at 35 weeks gestation. For me, my twins were born during this week.

One of my twins spent a week in the NICU, and the other spent two days in the continuing care nursery—a level above the NICU—before joining us at home. My argument is that because twin pregnancies are shorter than single pregnancies, you should plan ahead in case one or both of your infants need a longer hospital stay.

An Induction Story of Vaginal & Preterm Twin Birth

You can have a vaginal birth for your twins. This is the course of action I decided to take, as I have said. I'll tell you about the birth of my twins in this section. I chose to give birth to my twins vaginally because I thought the recovery after giving birth would be simpler. In addition, a friend of mine gave birth to her twins naturally.

Having this knowledge gave me greater confidence to attempt a vaginal birth with my twins. I reasoned that I might as well forego having surgery if I could avoid it. Despite being so frequent, a C-section is still a significant surgery that involves cutting you open. Having said that, my greatest worry was giving birth to twin A and then needing to undergo a C-section to deliver twin B.

When deciding whether to give birth to your own twins, it is a significant factor to take into account. To proceed with a vaginal birth, your twins must also cooperate and be facing down; at the very least, twin A must be head down.

Twins and Water Breaking

As previously said, at about 1:30 am, my water broke while I was sound asleep. At this point, I was 35.5 weeks pregnant. I was advised to visit the hospital when I called my doctor's office.

I was not experiencing any contractions throughout this period. The staff linked me up to a monitor when we got to the hospital to check if I was having contractions.

Though I was experiencing them, I wasn't feeling them. I was barely 3 cm dilated, and they weren't that close together.

Stated differently, I was not prepared to begin pressing.

The issue was that, if your water breaks, it's usually recommended that your baby be delivered within 24 hours because failing to do so raises the danger of infection. I was assigned a room and spent the entire day in the hospital, waiting for labor to begin on its own. The good news is that I felt very at ease throughout this period.

But regrettably, my labor did not advance quickly enough, so Pitocin was administered. I will simply say that the Pitocin helped me get from point A to point B in labor quite rapidly. Pitocin was administered, and the contractions were extremely strong.

In contrast, my singleton arrived entirely spontaneously, and I never had contractions as strong as I had when using pitocin. You will still feel a great deal of pressure and considerable discomfort even after receiving an epidural. You will eventually have an intense impulse to push as well.

<u>What Is the Length of a Twin's Birth?</u>

The time it takes to deliver your twins will vary, just like with other births. When you get to the hospital, you can already be in an advanced stage of labor and give birth quickly. Alternatively, it's possible that, similar to me, your water breaks and you have to wait a long time for it to be time to go.

Furthermore, a C-section may be an emergency or planned procedure. All of this indicates that there is a wide variation in the amount of time that passes between your arrival at the hospital and the birth of your twins. They might not be born for 48 hours or just a few hours.

I would also like to talk about how far apart twins are usually born. My twins were delivered vaginally, and they were not unusually born 25 minutes apart.

You should anticipate having twins born vaginally ranging from ten minutes to many hours apart. In contrast, you should anticipate having your twins delivered within a few minutes of one another if you undergo a C-section.

Recuperated after giving birth to twins

I would also like to provide a few observations about your twin postpartum healing. This is significant since I was unprepared for the healing process my body would undergo.

There is a lot of attention focused on your unborn child's health when you are pregnant. Moms are frequently completely ignored or treated as though they will recover quickly after giving birth.

It's crucial to maintain your health in order to care for your newborn twins. Having to deal with spinal headaches was one of the things I was not ready for.

One possible adverse consequence of receiving an epidural is having a spinal headache. I had the unpleasant situation of having to deal with them.

This meant that I would always get excruciating headaches, almost like a migraine, whenever I sat up straight. Caffeine and lying flat on my back were the only things that made a difference. It was really challenging to try to pump breast milk while traveling back and forth to the NICU. I wanted to be present for my twin kids, so I was filled with guilt.

My second issue after giving birth was a very tight neck. I pushed for one and a half hours, and during that time, I did something that really hurt my neck. My inability to sleep was impacted by this stiff neck pain. My neck hurt so much that it was excruciating for a few days after giving birth.

I didn't sleep at all for three days straight due to my neck pain, labor, and the time my water broke! That was something I had never experienced before, and it was really challenging.

I'm sharing these postpartum experiences with you to help you better understand some of the issues that may arise after your twins are born. The lesson here is to be ready for any unforeseen issues related to your postpartum recuperation.

In the event that your twin postpartum recovery is challenging, never forget that you must look after yourself in order to be ready to tend to your twins as soon as possible. If you're not feeling your best, don't feel bad about it.

I hope you feel more equipped to handle labor and delivery with twins now that you've read my tale of vaginal induction twin birth and maybe a twin C-section birth birth as well.

Essential oils can be a major help when you're trying to find out every natural method to make your home birth a little bit easier, whether you're running out of time or have plenty to spare before the big day! So, in what specific way may you use them to facilitate a home birth?

During your home birth, essential oils can help with anything from pain to fear and everything in between. They can greatly assist you by relieving your pain naturally, assisting with attention, and soothing you. To ensure the most straightforward home birth possible, continue reading to learn which ones to use and how to utilize them. Why give birth at home using essential oils?

You most likely picture your ideal home birth as a natural process involving the least amount of intervention.

This is made possible by essential oils, which provide you with a natural method of dealing with a multitude of issues. It basically makes things go more smoothly and reduces the likelihood that you may ask for pain relief during your home birth. Essential oils:

Unwind.

energize yourself

Aid in concentration

Reduce tension

Calm down

Reduce discomfort

They have been used for alternative medicine for hundreds of years, and they are still utilized for that purpose now (among so many other purposes).

I'm going to share with you one of the best-kept secrets about using essential oils to facilitate the simplest home birth possible.

There is an essential oil for every part of your home birth, whether it is to calm you down or to reduce your pain.

How to use essential oils for an easier home birth

There are many methods for enjoying the benefits of essential oils during your home birth. Some of them include:

- **Diffusion**- Dropping 6-10 drops into an essential oil diffuser. This method is great for relieving stress and anxiety as well as keeping you focused and alert.

- **Massage oil**- Pain relief is the main benefit of making a massage oil. You can do this by diluting 15-30 drops of essential oil in a tbsp. of fractioned coconut oil (or another carrier oil). Mix well and massage into the back, sides, hips, thighs or anywhere on the body you feel pain.

- **Hot/cold compress**– You can make these by soaking a rag in a water/essential oil mixture. You can either use a hot compress (for sore muscles and joints) or a cold compress (to reduce swelling and control pain).

- **In your birthing tub/pool**– If you opt to have a water birth, you can utilize the benefits of essential oils by dropping 10-20 drops of essential oil into your birthing tub.

Here are the top 7 best essential oils to make your home birth easier.

1. Eucalyptus Globulus for home birth

Eucalyptus oil has natural antiseptic, analgesic, and energizing properties that make it a must have for your home birth.

It aids in an easier home birth because it:

- **Relieves stress and anxiety.** Stress management is important for a home birth because it is an extremely stressful time in a mommas life.

- **Helps manage pain** using its main component, 1,8 Cineole, which accounts for up to 90% of the contents of Eucalyptus oil. . When inhaled, Eucalyptus oil has been shown to significantly decrease VAS (Visual Analog Scale) pain scores during labor.

- **Keeps your blood pressure in check.**High blood pressure (hypertension) is an extremely dangerous condition (especially during a home birth.) Eucalyptus oil has been proven to notably lower both systolic and diastolic blood pressure just by inhaling the aroma.

Set a stress-free, uplifting, and energizing environment, while also relieving your pain, by diffusing Eucalyptus Globulus in your birthing room.

Stress and fear are often associated with pain so reducing your stress in theory, reduces pain as well.

You can also use Eucalyptus oil in a topical pain reliever by creating a massage oil. It works even better when mixed half and half with Peppermint oil, which brings me to the next oil on my list.

2. Peppermint oil for home birth

Peppermint oil is an extremely versatile oil and a vital component to natural home birth because of all the beneficial properties it carries.

Peppermint essential oil can help to ease a home birth because it:

- **Eases pain** both topically and through inhalation.

- **Relieves nausea and vomiting** by simply inhaling the oil straight from the bottle or diffusing it into the air.

- **Increases focus and concentration** so you can keep your mind off your fear and pain.

- **Energizes your mind and body–** Birth is a tiresome process and takes a toll on your body as well as your energy level. *Diffusing Peppermint oil in your birth room gives you the energy and vitality you need to keep going!*

Peppermint has been shown to reduce pain in home birth through topical application thanks to the cooling and anti-inflammatory properties in its main component, Menthol.

3. Chamomile oil for home birth

Extremely calming and sedative-like, this oil acts as a *natural stress and pain reliever* upon inhalation.

No wonder it's one of the most recommended oils for a home birth.

Choose between both Roman and German Chamomile. They each have numerous benefits [that you may not be aware of] that make them perfect for helping you achieve the easiest home birth possible.

Chamomile aids in an easier home birth because it:

- **Relieves nausea and vomiting**- Stop these common symptoms associated with natural childbirth by inhaling it straight from the bottle or blending it with Peppermint, Ginger, and Lavender to maximize the anti-nausea benefits.

- **Naturally boosts mood**– Chamomile carries natural mood enhancing qualities that give you a positive, happy, and optimistic outlook.

- **Acts as a topical anti-inflammatory and analgesic-** Great in Sits baths or in the birthing tub to relieve any swelling and pain. You can also blend with a carrier oil along with other pain-relieving oils and massage into the skin to receive these benefits.

4. Geranium Essential oil for home birth

The sweet floral aroma carried by geranium is both grounding and restorative. It is well known for promoting emotional wellness, making it perfect for your home birth.

Geranium makes home birth easier by using it's:

- ***extremely potent*** **antiseptic, analgesic, and antispasmodic**

properties, all which aid in easier home birth.

- **grounding quality.** Geranium relieves both nervous anxiety and fear upon inhalation so diffusing it for this purpose is best.

- **strong aphrodisiac properties**. This makes it perfect for an orgasmic birth because the sheer scent of it can boost libido and put you in the mood.

Geranium can very well be used on its own during home birth but when mixed with Lavender and Rose oil, it creates a perfect ***home birth blend*** full of antiseptic, pain relieving, and mood boosting qualities sure to give you the home birth you imagined.

5. Lavender Essential oil for home birth

You knew it was coming! This is an all-around beneficial essential oil, well-known for its stress relieving and sleep-inducing benefits.

It is an absolutely perfect essential oil to make for an easier home birth for everyone involved.

Lavender works in a variety of ways by

- **Relieving pain**- It's been proven to ease aches and pains in studies.
- **Calming the mind and body**- Reduces stress and anxiety associated with

your fears of pain and thoughts of what is to come by relaxing you.

- **Reducing the risk of perineal tears because** of the relaxing effect it has on the body.

Inhale the exotic aroma of Lavender essential oil and let it take you to a happy, painless, and empowering place for the most amazing and natural experience of your life.

Tip: *Lavender essential oil is also perfect for perineal tears or lacerations postpartum. Just use it by dropping a few drops of Lavender oil in your sits bath along with a few drops of Chamomile. This not only helps heal the* *perineum but also relieves pain and inflammation.*

6. Clary Sage oil for home birth

Clary sage is by far the most beneficial oil to have next to you during your home birth. It is thought to help the uterine, respiratory, and muscular system during labor.

Clary sage should be avoided during pregnancy because it causes uterine contractions which can induce labor. That is the very reason it is so important during birth and delivery.

Clary sage has a lot of benefits that can make your home birth easier,

- **It speeds up delivery** by increasing oxytocin levels which, in turn, make contractions more productive.

- **It relieves pain through massage** because of its antiseptic properties. When you begin to feel contractions, massage a mixture of clary sage and carrier oil into your lower abdomen.

- **Promotes relaxation** during childbirth which can also speed up the process.

- **Regulates blood pressure** by relaxing the veins and arteries allowing blood to flow normally. It could also be attributed to its anti-inflammatory properties by reducing swelling and inflammation.

7. Grapefruit oil for home birth

With its deliciously citrus aroma, it's no surprise this essential oil made it on the list. This oil is perfect for labor and delivery as well as post partum.

The addition of Grapefruit essential oil can help make your home birth easier in various ways.

- **By encouraging happy vibes** in the room, brightening the air, and letting you release all negative feelings and have a positive outlook.

- **By relieving stress and anxiety** with its fruity uplifting scent.

- **By helping you fight fatigue.** It has natural energy boosting qualities that help you keep going when all your energy would normally be drained. As soon as you begin to feel any negative feelings or start to get worn out then you know it's time to pull out your Grapefruit essential oil.

Tip: *If you feel any baby blues after giving birth, this is the most beneficial oil to use because it helps you fight depression by naturally lifting your spirits and making you feel happy.*

Home birth blends

Certain oils blend well with each other and others not so well. Here are 3 blends perfect for making your home birth easier, PLUS they smell great together!

Home birth blend #1

These three oils together create a lovely floral aroma that will fill the birthing room with passion, a sense of calm and peace while also relieving pain and uplifting your spirit.

Diffuser Blend:

- 5 drops of Geranium
- 3 drops of Rose
- 5 drops of Lavender
-

Massage oil:

1 Tbsp. of fraction coconut oil or other carrier oil mixed with

- 10 drops Geranium
- 10 drops Lavender
- 7 drops Rose

Home birth blend #2

The fruity mint serenity created by the combination of Peppermint, Eucalyptus, and Grapefruit work together to lift your mood, help you focus, and also relieve labor pain. It also decreases stress, regulates blood pressure, and relieves inflammation.

Diffuser blend:

- 6 drops of Peppermint

- 4 drops of Eucalyptus Globulus
- 2 drops Grapefruit

Massage oil:

1 Tbsp. of carrier oil mixed with

- 12 drops of Peppermint
- 8 drops of Eucalyptus Globulus
- 6 drops of Grapefruit

Home Birth blend #3

This blend is specifically to support the relief of contraction pain and help make for a quicker labor. Either diffuse it at the beginning of labor or as soon as you start to feel labor pain. You can also massage into the abdomen, temples, neck, or the bottoms of feet to feel relief.

Diffuser Blend:

- 6 drops Clary Sage
- 4 drops Lavender
- 5 drops Geranium

Massage oil:

1 tbsp. of carrier oil mixed with

- 12 drops Clary Sage
- 8 drops Lavender
- 10 drops Geranium

Interactive: Birth Story Journal

- Space to document labor and delivery experiences

Chapter 8

Postpartum Recovery and Care

Your postpartum recovery schedule will be unique from other mothers' since it mostly depends on the nature of your childbirth experience.

According to medical professionals, recovery from a normal delivery—a vaginal birth without tearing—can take up to three weeks, but in my experience and in speaking with other mothers, this isn't always the case.

Whatever their type of labor and delivery, most moms begin to feel more like themselves at the 6-week mark after giving birth.

Furthermore, even while you might begin to feel more like yourself, postpartum recovery is not yet complete.

Recovery and Postpartum Care In the Initial Six Weeks Following Delivery

Your postpartum recovery plan should center around taking it easy on yourself to avoid infection and attempting to spend as much time as possible bonding with your baby during the first six weeks of life.

Mama, nevertheless, please don't overlook yourself!

INCLUDED IN YOUR EARLY POSTPARTUM RECOVERY PLAN SHOULD BE THE FOLLOWING:

AFTERPARTUM BLEEDING

You will suffer severe bleeding during the postpartum period, regardless of the type of labor you had (yeah, it's as great as it sounds, hehe).

Your body may decide to bleed for two weeks or go through six weeks of menstruation.

Thank goodness for mother nature, one never knows! The good news is that your bleeding will eventually stop, even if it takes longer.

Managing the excessive bleeding should be part of your early postpartum recovery plan so that you may feel comfortable and not worry about leaking.

(That's the LAST thing you have to worry about as you get used to being a new mother and/or host guests who want to see your kid).

THIS IS YOUR HEAVY BLEEDING POSTPARTUM RECOVERY PLAN:

To ensure that the maternity pads stay in place, choose up the long, thick pads WITH wings.

Additionally, you will need disposable mesh underwear (believe me, don't use your regular underwear) or old panties (yeah, I shudder too) that you don't want to get stained and discard later.

The most important thing is to be comfortable during the heaviest stage of your postpartum bleeding, so make sure you have your favorite pregnancy nightie or loose fitting leggings on hand.

To ensure that there are no leaks while you sleep, place a mattress protector pad on your bed.

POSTPARTUM CARE REQUIREMENTS

You are now aware of how to manage bleeding after giving birth, but what other necessities should your postpartum recovery plan include?

Now, let's review those.

PERI-BOTTLES

Mothers, you must get some peri bottles and put one in each of your restrooms.

Lightly mist your lady bits after adding lukewarm water to your bottle.

In addition to making me feel cleaner—which is such a great feeling—doing this helped me actually urinate after giving birth, which may be difficult even when you feel the need to go to the bathroom because of your swelling lower body.

Since my postpartum recuperation, I've spotted a peri bottle that I will ABSOLUTELY be picking up the next time around. It's called the Mom Washer, which is a fitting moniker, in my opinion. additionally, it functions effectively when the bottle is tipped upside down and features a curved spout that sprays water pleasantly.

COMFORTABLE WEAR

Mama, pull on your best pregnancy jeans and keep on dressing!

Despite what the media would have us believe, postpartum healing is not something that occurs in a matter of two weeks.

Okay, so just give yourself a break.

To ensure that you don't have to worry about anything during the first few weeks after giving birth, have your favorites cleaned and ready to go.

ITEMS FOR NURSING

You'll require many nursing bras.

Moreover, you want to get some nursing pads in case your baby leaks milk; the last thing you want is to show off a wet shirt to guests.

Basically, choose nursing supplies that you believe will be comfortable for YOU.

That is the objective.

Cozy, as you give yourself time to mend and give your darling new baby a hug.

(In my opinion, that is a really reasonable postpartum recovery plan for the first several weeks!)

Before I forget, don't forget to pick up a breastfeeding pillow. These are great for supporting the infant during breastfeeding or for simply lounging around with them on you.

GET THE STOL SOFTTENERS.

An essential component of your postpartum healing regimen will be stool softeners.

Why?

Because it will take some time for you to return to your previous level of regularity, whatever that means to you!

STORE A PAIN REMEDY ON AVAIL

Having your preferred painkillers on hand is crucial to your postpartum recovery plan because, mama, you will be sore.If you are breastfeeding, make sure it is safe for you to take.

GIVE BREASTFEEDING A BREAK TO YOURSELF

Mama, while you get used to being a new mother, a lot is going on.Give yourself a break if things don't go according to plan if you intend to breastfeed.

I'm not saying it won't work; just remember to take each day as it comes and that breastfeeding isn't always as simple as people think.

Too many of my mom friends have expressed worry about breastfeeding, and I believe that this can impede a quick recovery after giving birth.

Thus, be gentle with yourself.

WRAP POSTPARTUM BELLY

I didn't know that I should definitely get a belly wrap to help support and remind my abs of their proper place when I was postpartum.I really regret doing this!

My belly still needs to be flattened, and I've been postpartum for a while.(I promise not to make that error again!)

If you plan to have a C-section, a belly wrap is also an essential part of your postpartum recovery regimen.

A Sitz Bath Needs to Be a Part of Your Postpartum Rehabilitation Strategy

Do you know what a postpartum sitz bath is?

If not, you should absolutely include it in your postpartum recovery schedule!

Please, though, consult your doctor or midwife before taking a postpartum sitz bath.

It's one of those postpartum recovery strategies that many mothers suggest since it's both calming and restorative.

It also feels so wonderful.

Describe the SiTZ bath.

A postpartum sitz bath consists of submerging your lady bits into a little amount of warm water that has been infused with anti-inflammatory, healing, and pain-relieving substances.

(If using cold water makes you feel better, it's acceptable for some mothers to prefer to do so!)

In summary, that's a postpartum sitz bath. The idea is that it might hasten your recuperation from giving birth, and I have a feeling you'll do whatever it takes to achieve that!

A SITZ BATH: HOW DO YOU TAKE IT?

Either purchase an over-the-toilet sitz bath or put your ingredients to a small tub filled with water just deep enough to submerge your lady parts.

My entire body hurt, so I couldn't even consider lowering myself into the bathtub; I was afraid I wouldn't be able to get out again.

What you'll need is as follows:

✓Epsom Salts: An all-natural substance, epsom

salt will minimize swelling and provide a mild

cleansing, hence lowering the likelihood of infection.

Lavender: Add some essential oil of lavender to your sitz bath. Why? Due to its reputation as a natural antibacterial, lavender will ease your mind as you recover.

 Witch Hazel: This remedy has a long history of using its anti-infection and anti-inflammatory properties. It also relieves itching in the affected area. If you have extremely sensitive areas, the last thing you want to do is aggravate them. Look for witch hazel without alcohol.

Before you start the sitz bath, make sure all the components are thoroughly dissolved in the water.

Your Home-Based Postpartum Recovery Strategy

PLANNING MEALS AND FRIZZER MEALS

Make sure to prepare some meals for the freezer before giving birth if you are still pregnant.

Third trimester is an excellent time to work on list items, hehe!

When you're healing after giving birth, there's nothing better than taking out a prepared meal and warming it up.

Ask your husband and friends to assist prepare meals if you are currently postpartum and haven't frozen any.

When the meals in your freezer run out, you'll have to start meal planning again, but for now, you have this small infant who needs all of your care.

ALLOT of TIME FOR SELF-CARE.

Utilizing a postpartum sitz bath is one method to begin practicing self-care as you heal from giving birth.

However, you also need to make other time for yourself.

It can be pampering yourself with an extra-long, hot shower or napping while your partner watches the child.

Whatever makes you feel wonderful has to be done.

ASK FOR ASSISTANCE WHEN YOU NEED IT DURING YOUR POSTPARTUM RECOVERY.

One of the things that is, in my opinion, most underappreciated in postpartum recovery is asking friends and family for assistance.

Mothers are incapable of acknowledging when they need assistance.

The people closest to us want to help us; sometimes they're only waiting for us to ask for it, that's what we need to recognize.

So, during the first several weeks, have your mother or sister stay with you.

Get buddies to assist clean, or hire a cleaner.

For the first several weeks, at the very least, have your spouse prepare the meals and snacks.

And don't worry, you're still an amazing mother because you recently gave birth to a beautiful newborn!

SET AWAY YOUR HOUSEWORK TROUBLE

Please don't worry about the chores if, for whatever reason, you are unable to ask for assistance!

For once in your life, you won't be judged by others based on how tidy or untidy your home is.

So, make use of it.

Your postpartum recovery plan's goal should not include worrying about housework—rather, it should be to relax and enjoy your adorable infant!

You'll go back to it, so in the interim, unwind.

Interactive: Postpartum Health Checklist

- *Personalized checklist for postpartum care*

Chapter 9

Caring for Your Twins

How to Survive Newborn Twins

Let's be honest, caring for newborn twins is a lot of work. But, with a few tricks up your sleeve, it will be easier to survive. And, the good thing is, that even though it's tough, this is just a phase in yours and your twins' life.

Without further ado, let's get to the top tips for surviving life with newborn twins.

Newborn Twins Schedule

Before we get into the top hacks for surviving newborn twins, it's important you have an understanding of what to expect for a schedule with two newborns at home.

The reality is that newborn babies do not have a strict schedule that they follow. The first six weeks with your twins might end up feeling like a blur.

But, the good news is that newborns sleep A LOT! Most of the time newborns wake up, eat, and go back to sleep shortly after they are done with their feed.

On top of that, often twins are born on the early side. The earlier they are born the more sleep you can expect from them during their first few weeks of life.

As far as feeding, your babies will likely need to eat about every two hours. Sometimes this will be at the same time and sometimes your newborn twins will eat at different times.

The first 6 weeks with your twins will be an on demand type feeding schedule. With two babies to look after, it can feel overwhelming. But, you will survive and get through it.

One of the key things to work on during this time is teaching your twins cues for sleeping. You can do this by having the same routine when they are put to sleep.

An example of this would be swaddling your baby, holding and rocking them for a few minutes, then setting them down.

Surviving Nights With Newborn Twins

Besides introducing a baby bedtime routine, there are a few ways you could go for tackling a newborn twins sleep schedule at night.

One way to handle it is to rotate who takes care of the babies each night. This way every other night someone is getting a full night of sleep in the house.

This option is attractive because you know you will get sleep every other night. A negative (maybe?) is having to sleep in separate beds during this time.

A second option is to work in shifts. One person sleeps for a certain block of time at night, while the other parent cares for the twins. Then, they switch.

This option is nice because you know you will get your sleep, but the negative is you and your partner might not see each other much depending on your jobs and schedule.

A third option is to pick one baby to care for through the night. This is what me and my husband did.

We liked it because we had each other for support, but the downside was temporarily not being able to get a full night's sleep.

Taking Care of Twins When You're Alone

If you are going to be a single parent with newborn twins, handling nighttime is tricky.

If you can afford it, I would definitely look into hiring a night nurse. Since this is expensive, it doesn't have to be every night. But, it will be nice to get a break at least a couple nights a week.

It is also not a bad idea to look into this option for couples who are expecting twins. It will be a welcome break to have help at night once in a while. If I did it all over again, I would probably go this route.

Whatever strategy you choose for surviving newborn twins at night, you should definitely decide on what you think will work best for your situation before your twins are born.

If you start implementing it and it's just not working, you know there are other options to pursue.

How to Survive Breastfeeding Newborn Twins

As far as feeding your newborns, there will be differences in your goals and the help you can receive if you are exclusively breastfeeding twins versus if you are planning to formula feed them.

Additionally, there is always the possibility you are doing a combination of feeding them breast milk and formula.

If you do end up breastfeeding your twins, first of all, way to go! That is HARD work. Personally, I did a combination of pumping for my twins and using formula to supplement.

But, I do have breastfeeding experience because I breastfed my singleton through the first year. Since I had my singleton after my twins, I now know some pointers to help make breastfeeding newborn twins a little bit easier.

One thing that is important to understand if you are exclusively breastfeeding twins, is that you will have to be the one caring for them more often.

This is just natural because you need to breastfeed or pump for every feed, in order to produce enough breast milk. This means at night it will be harder to get a break.

One tip is you could plan pumping sessions and have whoever is around to help you wake up and feed the pumped breast milk. Even if it's just a couple nights a week to get a break and some sleep.

The other thing that's important to understand, is that sometimes during the newborn phase your twins will eat at the same time and sometimes they will eat at different times.

I recommend offering a feeding to both twins, if possible, even when only one of them is hungry. Sometimes this will work out in your favor and sometimes it won't.

At the end of the day, you will end up mastering breastfeeding a single baby and tandem breastfeeding your twins.

Bottle Feeding Newborn Twins

If you are pumping or formula feeding, you will be able to get a little bit more help with feeding your twins.

When help is around, take up any and all that you have. Feeding your twins a bottle is a somewhat easy task you can ask people around the house to help with.

An important thing to do with bottle feeding twins is mastering quick bottle preparation.

You will also need to figure out how to feed twins by yourself. This was something I stressed about the first 6 weeks because I did have help.

I was very worried about what would happen when my mom left, I had no idea how I would handle my newborns alone.

But, guess what? You just figure it out, because you have to. I did practice tandem feeding them their bottles while she was still staying with me. This allowed me to feel slightly less stressed about being alone.

How to Get Out of the House With Newborn Twins

Trying to find a change of scenery besides your own house when you have newborn twins is difficult, especially if you are caring for them alone.

The best thing I did was take a walk any day that was nice enough when I was home on maternity leave.

The reason I liked this was the stress level was low. If one of them cried, I was outside and not really bothering anyone.

Plus, I was still close to home. If I had forgotten anything, I could just run home and get it.

I think it's a good goal to have to go outside and take a walk as much as possible with your newborn babies.

How to Run Errands With Twins

There will be times that you want to do more than take a walk with your babies. And, it is possible to do this.

The best way to go about this is have your diaper bag packed for twins and ready to go and in the car. Plan for only one or two errands and know exactly what you need to do.

Secondly, plan to leave as soon as your twins have finished a feeding to maximize your time. This is not to say you can't feed your twins when you are out. But, if you don't want to worry about that then, this is a good way to do it.

Personally, I found it easiest to just go out for short trips. Also, I would go to places that were close by, since newborns need to eat often.

Newborns also sleep a lot, so running short errands can actually be okay. Most of the time or maybe even the whole time, they will just be asleep.

I do think starting with small trips are good because you get practice. You can see what it takes to get out of the house with twins. Then, you can build up to longer outings as you get a feel for what you can handle.

Tips for Surviving Newborn Twins

So, there you have it. Those are all my tips from sleeping to feeding to getting out of the house with newborn twins.

Before I go, here is a list to summarize the top tips for surviving newborn twins.

Introduce a baby bedtime or sleep routine.

Pick a strategy for handling your newborn twins at night, preferably before they are born.

Consider hiring a night nurse, especially if you will be caring for your twins alone.

Be prepared to feed newborn twins OFTEN. Whether you are breastfeeding or bottle feeding, having the correct supplies ready for feedings will help them go more smoothly.

Taking a walk is an easy way to get out of the house with newborn babies.

When running errands with twins, start with quick trips that are close to home.

I hope you are able to put some of these tips to good use.

Interactive: Twin Care Log

- Log for feeding, sleeping, and development

Chapter 10

How To Tell Identical Twins Apart

Wow, they look so much alike! How do you tell them apart?

Oh, that's easy. They dance differently.

Alright, that is a bit of a tongue in cheek answer to a question I get asked all the time. People always want to know how I can tell my identical twins apart.

I'm not wrong about the dancing thing. They do each have their own unique moves. But there are more ways than that.

While now I feel pretty confident in telling my daughters apart, one of my biggest worries during my twin pregnancy was that I wouldn't be able to. I think this is pretty normal. Fortunately, there are several systems you can use to tell your identical twins apart.

Try these when you are asking yourself How can you tell identical twins apart?

Telling twins apart is a fear that comes up for pretty much every twin mom. It doesn't matter if you are having identical girl twins like me, I have heard this fear about fraternal twins too. Babies look a lot alike, and in the sleep-deprived early crazy days you can confuse your boy twin for your girl twin.

The biggest thing to remember about telling identical twins apart is that you are their parents. You will learn every little difference between them. You just know your family.

To build your confidence, there are several things you can do.

Keep the Hospital Bands

Our hospital helped us out right from the start by putting the girls' bands on opposite wrists. This helped us know who was who at a glance. Of course, there was also the obvious fact that the bands had Baby A and Baby B on them. That helped too.

Try Some Nail Polish

Using polish on a nail is a great way to tell who is who. I painted the big toe of each girl in different colors. Babies like to suck on their hands, so I didn't want to put anything on their fingers, just in case.

And I wanted to put colors on each girl in case it scratched off one. This way we had two colors to rely on, not just one with color and one without.

The drawback to this method is in the middle of the night you might not be able to see your babies' toes, it did make me feel better knowing we had an additional identification method in place.

Assign Clothing Choices

An easy way to help in telling identical twin babies apart is color coding. We didn't necessarily assign one color to each boy. (We had too many blue items to make that practical.) But once one boy wore something, it was his. No switching allowed.

There were a few rules we followed. Given the choice of blue and non blue. One baby got everything with cats on it. These are just a couple of examples.

I know some twin moms who assigned one twin a color and the other got everything else. One could have solids and the other patterns. There are lots of ways to do it.

I would jot down the outfits every time I changed the boys. I didn't do anything fancy, but I was already writing down notes on eating and sleeping, so noting outfits wasn't hard. In a moment of panic, these notes were invaluable.

Note Physical Characteristics

Even in identical twins, there will be some physical differences. Identical twins do split from a single egg, but once they have split they each have their own unique experiences, even in the womb. As a result, they can have physical differences.

Things like freckles and moles are in different places. Birthmarks are usually unique between identical twins.

A big thing to check is the belly button. Everyone's belly button is unique. They are basically surgical scars, as every cut of the umbilical cord will be different. Physical differences between twins may be subtle, but you have plenty of time to study them during the hours of feedings in those first few weeks.

How To Tell Twins Apart in Pictures

Now that my boys are older I am confident I know who is who. They each have their own spark and personality, making it easier for me at least to tell them apart.

Pictures are a different issue. I think I can tell them apart in pictures but honestly, I have several where I am just guessing. (Remember a lot of newborns look alike, not just twins.) There are ways to combat that as well. Whatever system you choose, make sure to go over your pictures and write down who is in the picture. I think I will remember what outfits I assigned which baby, but already I know I am forgetting. It is well worth taking the time to label any pictures so in a few years you aren't wondering who is in your shots.

Differences in Identical Twins

Despite the name, identical twins are rarely 100% identical. Identicals have different fingerprints, belly buttons, and birthmarks. As they age more and more differences can appear, even when it comes to height.

How we grow and develop depends on both nature (our DNA) and nurture (our experiences). No two people share the same exact life experiences, not even identical twins. As a result, they will not be exactly the same. Identical twins might even have one left-handed twin and one right-handed!

As your twins grow and develop you will learn what makes each twin special. (Like having their own dance moves.)

Give Yourself Grace as a Twin Parent

There will be times when you mix up your twins. You will call them by the wrong name. This is so normal.

As a twin parent, I know I feel the pressure to make sure I recognize my daughters as individuals, not as a set. So I feel guilty when I mix them up! The truth is, they do look a lot alike. So at a glance, I might not be able to definitively say who is who, especially from behind.

But you will be able to tell your twins apart. Once I take that second to really look, I know exactly who I am talking to, regardless of anything else going on. And that recognition sets in earlier than you might think.

Give yourself some grace. It doesn't mean you don't love your babies, and it doesn't mean you only see them as a unit. It just means you're human.

You will be able to tell your twins apart. These systems can give you added reassurance that you know who is who. I think that is important for peace of mind. It is normal to call out the wrong name, and that doesn't make you a bad mom. You will know your babies.

Interactive session

write down the changes you've noticed so far in your twins and your personal method of identification if any or the method you got from this book

247

Conclusion

As you reach the end of this holistic guide to twin pregnancy, take a moment to reflect on the incredible journey you've embarked upon. Carrying twins is a unique and beautiful experience, filled with both challenges and joys. By embracing holistic practices, you've nurtured not only your physical health but also your emotional and spiritual well-being.

Throughout this book, we explored the importance of a balanced diet, mindful movement, and self-care. We've discussed the power of mindfulness, the benefits of prenatal yoga, and the value of a supportive community. Each of these practices plays a vital role in creating a nurturing environment for both you and your babies.

Remember, your journey doesn't end with the birth of your twins. Parenthood brings new adventures and opportunities for growth. Continue to prioritize your well-being, seek support when needed, and cherish the special bond you've already begun to form with your little ones.

As you move forward, may you carry with you the knowledge, tools, and confidence to embrace the beautiful chaos of twin motherhood. Celebrate every milestone, big or small, and know that you are never alone on this journey.

Thank you for allowing this book to be a part of your path. Wishing you a healthy, joyful, and fulfilling experience as you welcome your twins into the world.

Glossary of Terms

Antenatal Care: Regular medical check-ups during pregnancy to monitor the health of the mother and babies.

Chorionicity: Refers to the number of placentas in a twin pregnancy, important for determining potential risks.

Diastasis Recti: Separation of abdominal muscles during pregnancy, common in multiple pregnancies.

Folic Acid: A vital B-vitamin recommended during pregnancy to prevent neural tube defects.

Gestational Diabetes: A form of diabetes that develops during pregnancy, requiring special management.

Kegel Exercises: Exercises to strengthen the pelvic floor muscles, beneficial during and after pregnancy.

Monozygotic Twins: Identical twins formed from a single fertilized egg that splits into two.

Omega-3 Fatty Acids: Essential fats important for fetal brain development, found in fish and supplements.

Perinatal: The period shortly before and after birth, focusing on the health of the mother and babies.

Placenta: An organ that develops in the uterus during pregnancy, providing oxygen and nutrients to the fetus.

Preeclampsia: A pregnancy complication characterized by high blood pressure and potential organ damage.

Prenatal Vitamins: Supplements containing essential vitamins and minerals recommended during pregnancy.

Toxoplasmosis: An infection that can be harmful during pregnancy, often transmitted through certain foods or cat litter.

Twin-to-Twin Transfusion Syndrome (TTTS): A condition where identical twins share blood circulation unevenly, requiring medical attention.

Ultrasound: An imaging technique used to monitor the development of the fetus during pregnancy.

Frequently Asked Questions (FAQs)

Q: What are the nutritional requirements for a twin pregnancy?

A: Nutritional needs are higher in a twin pregnancy. Focus on a balanced diet rich in proteins, iron, folic acid, calcium, and omega-3 fatty acids. Consult your healthcare provider for personalized recommendations.

Q: How much weight should I expect to gain with twins?

A: Weight gain varies, but generally,

women carrying twins may gain between 35 to 45 pounds. Your healthcare provider can give personalized guidance based on your pre-pregnancy weight.

Q: What types of exercises are safe during a twin pregnancy?

A: Safe exercises include walking, swimming, and prenatal yoga. Always consult your doctor before starting any exercise regimen to ensure it's suitable for your condition.

Q: How can I manage stress during my twin pregnancy?

A: Mindfulness practices, such as meditation and deep breathing, along with prenatal yoga, can help reduce stress. Engaging in relaxing activities and connecting with support groups can also be beneficial.

Q: What are the signs of preterm labor in a twin pregnancy?

A: Signs include regular contractions, back pain, pelvic pressure, and changes in vaginal discharge. Contact your healthcare provider immediately if you experience any of these symptoms.

Q: How is labor different with twins?

A: Labor with twins may be different, including the potential for a cesarean delivery or different stages of labor for each twin. Discuss your birth plan and options with your healthcare provider.

Q: Can I breastfeed twins?

A: Yes, many mothers successfully breastfeed twins. Support from lactation consultants and using strategies like tandem nursing can be helpful.

Q: What are common postpartum concerns for mothers of twins?

A: Common concerns include fatigue, emotional adjustment, and physical recovery. Seeking support from family, friends, or postpartum doulas can be beneficial.

Q: How can I prepare for bringing home twins?

A: Prepare by setting up a comfortable nursery, arranging for extra help, and stocking up on essentials like diapers and clothing. Joining support groups for parents of multiples can provide valuable insights and support.

www.ingramcontent.com/pod-product-compliance
Lightning Source LLC
Chambersburg PA
CBHW051552250726
48653CB00004BA/1113